FIBER FUELED COOKBOOK FOR BEGINNERS

Plant-Based High fiber recipes for weight loss and maintenance and Health balance microbiome, nutrient-rich and gut friendly ingredients.

By

Sophia Roberts

TABLE OF CONTENT

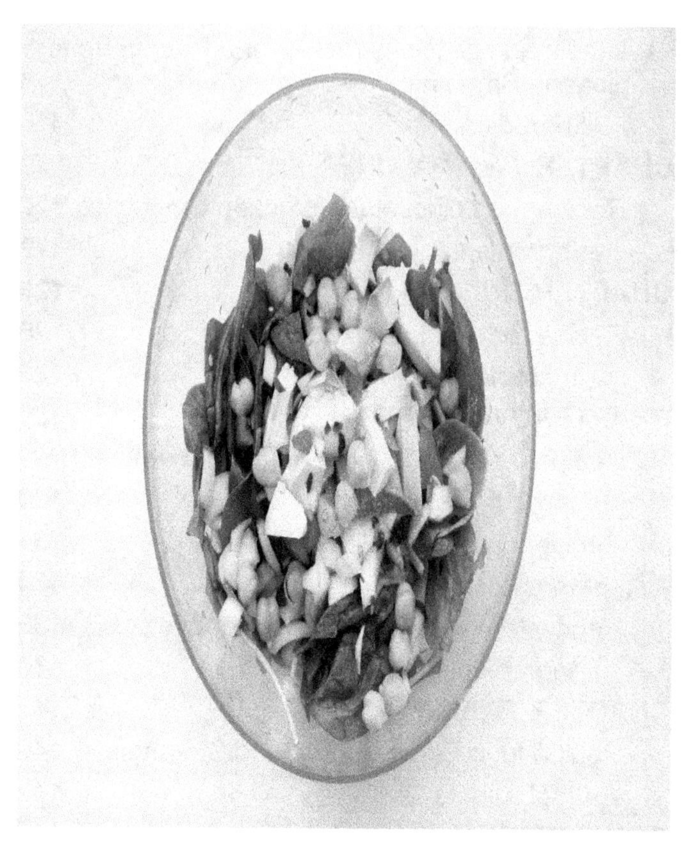

Introduction

In a world filled with countless diets and nutritional advice, there's one often-overlooked hero in the realm of wellness: fiber. It's not just a bland component of your meals; it's a potent catalyst for a healthier, more vibrant life. Welcome to the "Fiber Fueled Cookbook for Beginners," your passport to a culinary voyage that merges the joys of eating with the science of nourishing your body.

Fiber is the unsung champion of nutrition, known for its role in digestive health, weight management, and even its potential to reduce the risk of chronic diseases. This cookbook is your roadmap to unlocking the full potential of fiber-rich foods. Whether you're a novice in the kitchen or a seasoned chef, the recipes within these pages will inspire and delight your taste buds. Prepare to embark on a journey that transcends

salads and bran muffins.
From hearty breakfasts that kickstart your day to satisfying dinners that leave you nourished and fulfilled, our recipes are both delicious and simple to make. They showcase the vibrant colors, flavors, and textures of plant-based ingredients, proving that eating for health can also be a delightful gastronomic experience.

This cookbook, however, is more than just a collection of recipes.It's a guide that demystifies the world of fiber, providing you with the knowledge you need to make informed dietary choices. You'll discover how fiber promotes gut health, aids in weight management, and supports overall well-being. So, join us on this culinary adventure, where every dish is a celebration of flavor, health, and the transformative power of fiber. It's time to fuel your life with fiber. The "Fiber Fueled Cookbook for Beginners" is a culinary journey that empowers you to harness the incredible health benefits of fiber-rich foods while savoring delicious and easy-to-make recipes. In a world where dietary choices play a pivotal role in our well-being, this cookbook is your gateway to a healthier, more vibrant life. Let's embark on this exciting adventure together, exploring the wonders of fiber and discovering how it can transform your kitchen and your health.

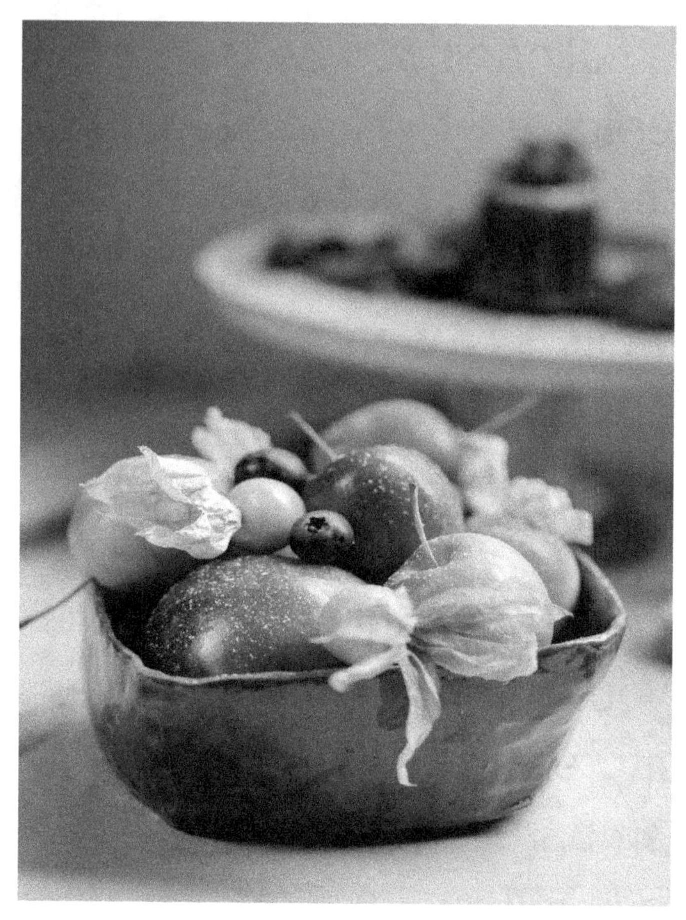

CHAPTER ONE

What is Fiber?

Fiber, often referred to as roughage or bulk, is a crucial component of plant-based foods that plays a fundamental role in our digestive health and overall well-being. Unlike other nutrients like carbohydrates, proteins, and fats, fiber is not digested or absorbed by the body. Instead, it passes through the digestive system largely intact, offering a multitude of health benefits.

There are two forms of dietary fiber: **soluble** and **insoluble**. Soluble fiber dissolves with water in the digestive tract to form a gel-like substance. It helps regulate blood sugar levels, lower cholesterol, and support a healthy gut by nourishing beneficial gut bacteria. On the other hand, insoluble fiber does not dissolve in water and adds bulk to stool, aiding in regular bowel movements and preventing constipation.

Fiber-rich foods are primarily found in fruits, vegetables, whole grains, legumes, nuts, and seeds. Consuming an ample amount of fiber is associated with numerous health advantages, including improved digestive function, weight management, and a reduced risk of chronic diseases such as heart disease, type 2 diabetes, and certain cancers.

Incorporating fiber into your diet is a powerful way to support your overall health, and this cookbook will guide you in creating delicious, fiber-packed meals that are not only nutritious but also satisfying to your taste buds.

Health benefits of fiber

Fiber is a dietary superhero, offering a treasure trove of health benefits that can transform your well-being. Here are some compelling reasons to make fiber-rich foods a fundamental part of your daily diet:

Digestive Health

 Fiber acts as nature's broom, promoting regular bowel movements and preventing constipation. It adds bulk to stool, making it easier to pass through the digestive tract while preventing common gastrointestinal issues.

Weight Management:

High-fiber foods tend to be filling and satisfying, helping to control appetite and reduce overall calorie intake. This can be a game-changer in achieving and maintaining a healthy weight.

Blood Sugar Control:

Soluble fiber, found in foods like oats and legumes, can slow the absorption of sugar, helping to stabilize blood sugar levels.

Heart Health:

Fiber-rich diets are linked to a reduced risk of heart disease. Soluble fiber helps lower LDL cholesterol levels, while insoluble fiber supports healthy blood pressure and reduces inflammation in the arteries.

Gut Microbiome Support:

Fiber nourishes beneficial gut bacteria, fostering a diverse and healthy microbiome. A balanced gut flora is associated with improved immune function and a decreased risk of digestive disorders.

Reduced Cancer Risk:

Some studies suggest that a high-fiber diet may lower the risk of certain cancers, such as colorectal cancer. Fiber aids in the removal of waste and toxins from the body, potentially reducing the exposure of cells to harmful substances.

Longevity:
 Research indicates that individuals who consume more fiber tend to live longer and enjoy a higher quality of life in their later years. The protective effects of fiber on various aspects of health contribute to increased longevity.

Incorporating fiber into your diet isn't just a smart choice; it's a delicious one too. With the Fiber Fueled Cookbook for Beginners, you can relish the culinary delights of fiber-rich foods while reaping the remarkable health benefits they offer. Elevate your health and savor the journey to a vibrant, fulfilling life with the power of fiber.

Fiber is a stalwart ally when it comes to promoting gut health. It acts as a potent guardian, fostering an environment in your digestive system that supports both your physical and mental well-being. Here's how fiber accomplishes this:

Feeding Beneficial Bacteria:

Fiber serves as the preferred food source for the trillions of beneficial bacteria residing in your gut. These microorganisms, collectively known as the gut microbiome, play a pivotal role in digestion, nutrient absorption, and immune function. When you consume fiber-rich foods, you're essentially nourishing these friendly microbes, allowing them to thrive and maintain a balanced ecosystem.

Producing Short-Chain Fatty Acids (SCFAs): As fiber is broken down by gut bacteria, it produces valuable byproducts called short-chain fatty acids (SCFAs). These SCFAs, like butyrate, acetate, and propionate, have been linked to numerous health benefits. They help maintain the integrity of the gut lining, reduce inflammation, and even support brain health.

Enhancing Regularity:

Insoluble fiber, found in foods like whole grains and vegetables, adds bulk to stool, making it easier to move through the digestive tract. This aids in regular and healthy bowel movements, preventing constipation and related discomfort.

Balancing Gut pH:

Fiber can help regulate the pH levels in the gut, creating an environment that's less hospitable to harmful bacteria. This pH balance is vital for a healthy gut microbiome.

By promoting a diverse and thriving community of beneficial bacteria, fiber helps reduce gut inflammation. Chronic inflammation in the gut is associated with various digestive disorders and can have broader health implications.

Incorporating fiber-rich foods into your diet is a surefire way to nurture your gut microbiome and lay the foundation for excellent digestive health. It's not just about what you eat; it's about cultivating a thriving ecosystem within you.

Fiber's importance in your weight reduction journey

Fiber plays a pivotal role in weight loss and healthy

weight management by offering a range of benefits that support your journey toward achieving and maintaining a healthy weight.

Here are 10 strong points highlighting the roles fiber plays in weight loss:

Enhanced Satiety:

Fiber-rich foods are often more filling and satisfying, helping you feel full for longer periods. This reduced hunger sensation can lead to decreased calorie intake.

Caloric Dilution:

Many high-fiber foods, like fruits and vegetables, are low in calories but high in volume. This means you can eat more of them while consuming fewer calories, making it easier to control your calorie intake.

Reduced Snacking:

Fiber helps stabilize blood sugar levels, preventing the rapid spikes and crashes that can lead to between-meal snacking on less healthy options.

Slower Digestion:

Fiber-rich foods take longer to digest, providing a sustained release of energy and reducing the urge to eat again shortly after a meal.

Decreased Absorption of Calories:

Soluble fiber can bind to some dietary fats and calories, reducing their absorption by the body and effectively lowering calorie intake.

Lower Energy Density:

Foods with high fiber content often have a lower energy density, meaning they provide fewer calories for the same volume of food. This promotes weight loss by encouraging the consumption of larger portions of low-calorie foods.

Gut Microbiome Balance:

Fiber nourishes beneficial gut bacteria, and a healthy gut microbiome is linked to improved metabolism and weight regulation.

Improved Hormonal Balance:

Fiber can influence the hormones that regulate appetite and satiety, helping you make healthier food choices and control your eating habits.

Long-Term Weight Maintenance:

A high-fiber diet is not just effective for weight loss; it also supports long-term weight maintenance by promoting healthier eating habits and reducing the likelihood of regaining lost weight.

Incorporating fiber-rich foods like whole grains, fruits, vegetables, legumes, and nuts into your daily diet

is a powerful strategy for achieving and sustaining a healthy weight. It's a natural, sustainable approach that can make a significant difference in your weight loss journey.

Benefits of fiber in weight maintenance:

Fiber is a potent ally in the realm of weight maintenance, serving as a valuable tool to help you sustain a healthy weight over the long term. Here's how fiber is instrumental in this endeavor:

Satiety and Appetite Control: High-fiber foods, such as fruits, vegetables, and whole grains, are known for their ability to create a sense of fullness and satiety. This helps you control your appetite, reduce overeating, and maintain portion control, crucial elements in maintaining your weight.

Stable Blood Sugar:

Fiber-rich foods have a slower impact on blood sugar levels due to their complex carbohydrates. This steadier rise and fall in blood sugar help prevent energy crashes and the subsequent cravings for high-calorie, sugary snacks that can lead to weight gain.

Reduced Risk of Weight Regain: After successful weight loss, many individuals struggle with weight regain. Fiber-rich diets can help prevent this by encouraging the consumption of nutrient-dense, filling foods that promote fullness and discourage overindulgence.

Healthy Microbiome:

A diet rich in fiber nourishes beneficial gut bacteria, contributing to a balanced and diverse gut microbiome. This balance is associated with improved metabolism and weight regulation.

Balanced Nutrient Intake:

Fiber-rich foods are often nutrient-dense, providing essential vitamins and minerals alongside their fiber content. This ensures that your body receives the necessary nutrients while managing your calorie intake.

Long-Term Sustainability:

Unlike fad diets or extreme restrictions, incorporating fiber into your diet is a sustainable and enjoyable approach to weight maintenance. It promotes a balanced and varied diet that can be maintained over time.

By making fiber a cornerstone of your dietary choices, you create a supportive environment for weight maintenance. It's a natural, wholesome, and effective strategy that not only helps you achieve your weight goals but also empowers you to maintain a healthy weight for years to come.

General benefits of fiber

Fiber is a remarkable and multifaceted component of your diet that supports overall well-being in several key ways:

Digestive Health:

Fiber is a digestive system champion. It promotes regular bowel movements, prevents constipation, and helps maintain a healthy gut environment. It's essential for the efficient processing and elimination of waste from the body.

Weight Management:

Fiber-rich foods are often low in calories but high in volume, making you feel full and satisfied. This helps control your appetite, reduce calorie intake, and support healthy weight management.

Blood Sugar Control:

Soluble fiber, found in foods like oats and legumes, can slow the absorption of sugar, helping to stabilize blood sugar levels.This is especially important for people who have diabetes or are at risk of developing it.

Heart Health:

 A high-fiber diet is linked to a reduced risk of heart disease. Soluble fiber helps lower LDL ("bad") cholesterol levels, while insoluble fiber supports healthy blood pressure and reduces inflammation in the arteries.

Gut Microbiome Balance:

Fiber nourishes beneficial gut bacteria, promoting a diverse and healthy gut microbiome. A balanced gut flora is associated with improved immune function and a decreased risk of digestive disorders.

Reduced Risk of Chronic Diseases: A fiber-rich diet is associated with a lower risk of chronic conditions such as type 2 diabetes, certain cancers (e.g., colon cancer), and obesity-related disease.

Reduced Inflammation: Fiber's impact on the gut microbiome and its production of short-chain fatty acids can help reduce inflammation throughout the body. Chronic inflammation is a significant driver of numerous disorders.

Improved Longevity: Research suggests that individuals who consume more fiber tend to live longer and enjoy a higher quality of life in their later years. The protective effects of fiber on various aspects of health contribute to increased longevity.

Incorporating a variety of fiber-rich foods, such as fruits, vegetables, whole grains, legumes, nuts, and seeds, into your daily diet is a simple and effective way to enhance overall well-being and contribute to a healthier, more vibrant life. It's not just about eating; it's about nourishing your body from the inside out.

CHAPTER TWO

Recipes

Chickpea and Spinach Curry:

Ingredients:

1 can chickpeas, drained and rinsed

1 onion, chopped

2 cloves garlic, minced

1 can diced tomatoes

2 cups fresh spinach

1 tbsp olive oil

1 tsp curry powder

1/2 tsp turmeric
Salt and pepper to taste

Directions:

Olive oil should be heated in a sizable pan at medium heat. Add the minced garlic and onions, and cook until softened.

Stir in curry powder and turmeric, cooking for another minute.

Add chickpeas and diced tomatoes with their juice.

Simmer for 15 to 20 minutes to let flavors blend.

Just before serving, stir in fresh spinach until wilted.

Season with salt and
pepper to taste. Serve over
brown rice.

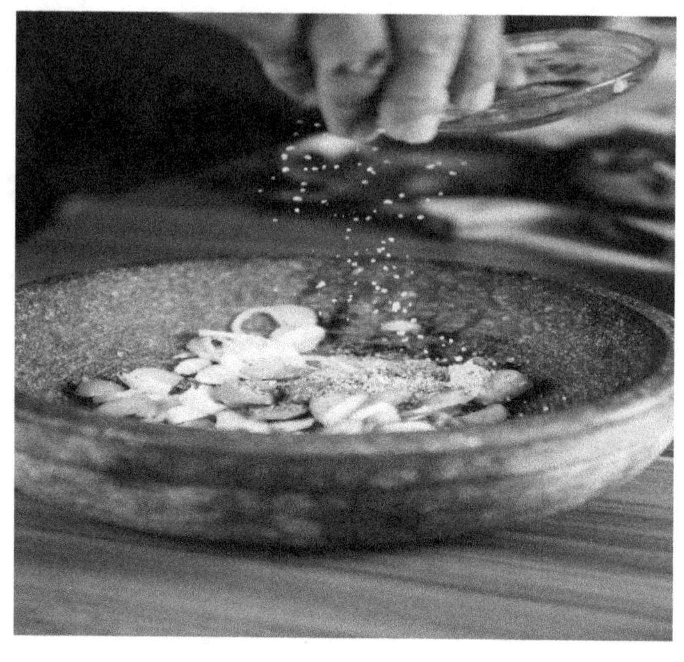

CHAPTER THREE

Bell peppers filled with black beans and quinoa

Ingredients:

4 bell peppers, any color

1 cup quinoa, cooked

1 can black beans, drained and rinsed

1 cup corn kernels (frozen or canned)

1 cup diced tomatoes

1 tsp cumin

Salt and pepper to taste

Directions:

Preheat your oven to 375°F (190°C).

Cut off the tops of the bell peppers and remove the seeds and membranes.

After 5 minutes of partial boiling in boiling water, drain the peppers.

In a bowl, combine cooked quinoa, black beans, corn, diced tomatoes, cumin, salt, and pepper.

Stuff the quinoa mixture inside each bell pepper.

Place the stuffed peppers in a baking dish, cover with foil, and bake for 25-30 minutes, until peppers are tender.

CHAPTER FOUR

Mediterranean Chickpea Salad:

Ingredients:

2 cans chickpeas, drained and rinsed
1 cucumber, diced
1 cup cherry tomatoes, halved
1/2 red onion, thinly sliced
1/4 cup kalamata olives, pitted and sliced
Juice of 1 lemon
2 tbsp olive oil
Fresh parsley, chopped, for garnish

Vegan feta cheese
(optional)
Directions:
In a large bowl, combine
chickpeas, cucumber,
cherry tomatoes, red onion,
and kalamata olives.
In a small bowl, whisk
together lemon juice and
olive oil, then drizzle over
the salad.
Combine all ingredients and
sprinkle with the fresh
parsley.
If desired, crumble vegan
feta cheese on top.

CHAPTER FIVE

Sweet Potato and Black Bean
Tacos:

2 large sweet potatoes,
peeled and diced
1 can black beans, drained
and rinsed
1 avocado, sliced
Whole wheat tortillas
Lime-cilantro dressing:
Juice of 2 limes
1/4 cup fresh cilantro,
chopped
1 clove garlic, minced
2 tbsp olive oil
Salt and pepper to taste

Preheat your oven to 425°F
(220°C)
Add salt, pepper, and olive
oil to the sweet potato
cubes and toss.
Roast for 25-30 minutes
until tender.
In a small bowl, whisk
together lime juice, cilantro,
garlic, olive oil, salt, and
pepper.
Warm the tortillas, then fill
with roasted sweet
potatoes, black beans,

avocado slices, and drizzle
with lime-cilantro dressing.

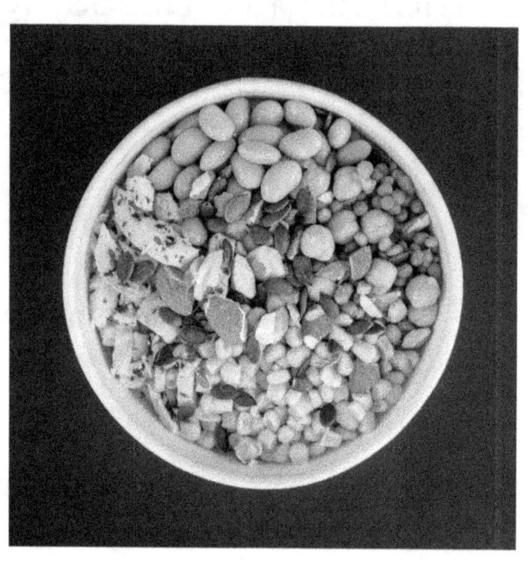

CHAPTER SIX

Three-Bean Chili:

1 can kidney beans, drained and rinsed

1 can black beans, drained and rinsed

1 can pinto beans, drained and rinsed

1 can diced tomatoes

1 onion, chopped

2 cloves garlic, minced

1 red bell pepper, chopped

1 green bell pepper, chopped

2 tbsp chili powder

1 tsp cumin
1 tsp paprika
Salt and pepper to taste
Vegetable broth

Directions:

Olive oil should be heated in a sizable pan at medium heat. Add the minced garlic and onions, and cook until softened
Cook for a couple more minutes after adding the diced bell peppers.
Stir in chili powder, cumin, and paprika.
Add kidney beans, black beans, pinto beans, and

diced tomatoes. Add
enough vegetable broth to
reach your desired chili
consistency.
Simmer, stirring from time to
time, for at least thirty
minutes.
Season with salt and
pepper to taste. Serve hot.

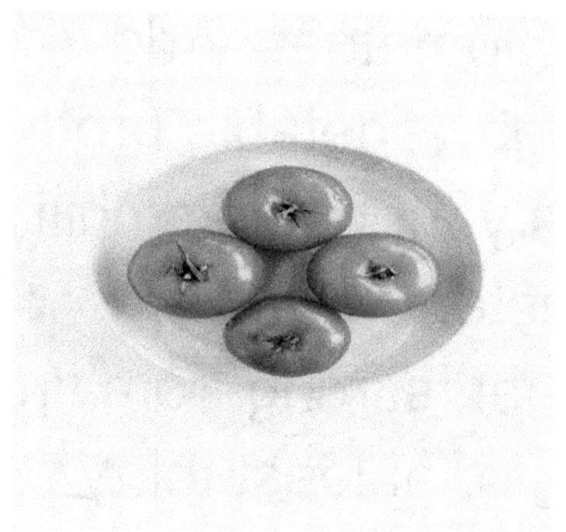

CHAPTER SEVEN

Berry and Chia Seed Breakfast
Bowl:

One cup of mixed berries,
such as blueberries,
raspberries and
strawberries
2 tbsp chia seeds
1/2 cup unsweetened
almond milk
1 tbsp honey or maple
syrup (optional)
Sliced almonds for garnish

Directions:

In a bowl, mix the chia seeds and almond milk. Stir well and let it sit for 15 minutes or until it thickens. Top with mixed berries, drizzle with honey or maple syrup if desired, and garnish with sliced almonds.

CHAPTER EIGHT

Lentil and Vegetable Soup:

Ingredients:

One cup of rinsed and dried
green or brown lentils
1 onion, chopped
2 carrots, diced
2 celery stalks, chopped
4 cups vegetable broth
1 can diced tomatoes
2 tsp dried thyme
Salt and pepper to taste

Directions:

In a large pot, sauté onions, carrots, and celery in a bit of vegetable broth until softened.

Add the diced tomatoes, lentils, vegetable broth, thyme, salt, and pepper. Lentils should be cooked for 25 to 30 minutes or until soft.

CHAPTER NINE

Spinach and Chickpea Salad:

Ingredients:

4 cups fresh spinach leaves
1 can chickpeas, drained and rinsed
1 red bell pepper, diced
1/4 cup red onion, thinly sliced
Balsamic vinaigrette dressing

Directions:

In a large bowl, combine spinach, chickpeas, diced red bell pepper, and sliced red onion.

Toss to coat, then drizzle
with balsamic vinaigrette
dressing.

CHAPTER TEN

Roasted Veggie and Quinoa Bowl:

Ingredients:

1 cup quinoa, cooked
Assorted roasted
vegetables (e.g., bell
peppers, zucchini, broccoli,
cherry tomatoes)
1/4 cup hummus
Lemon tahini dressing (mix
tahini, lemon juice, garlic,
and water)

Directions:

Bake the veggies until they
are soft.

In a bowl, layer cooked
quinoa, roasted vegetables,
and a dollop of hummus.
Drizzle with lemon tahini
dressing.

CHAPTER ELEVEN

Black Bean and Corn Salsa:

Ingredients:

1 can black beans, drained
and rinsed
1 cup corn kernels (fresh or
frozen)
1 red onion, finely chopped
1 red bell pepper, diced
1/4 cup fresh cilantro,
chopped
Juice of 2 limes
Salt and pepper to taste

Directions:

In a large bowl, combine black beans, corn, chopped red onion, diced red bell pepper, and fresh cilantro. Drizzle with lime juice and season with salt and pepper. Before serving, give it a good stir and let it cool for a few hours.

CHAPTER TWELVE

Roasted Vegetable Stir Fry with Peanut Sauce:

Ingredients:

For the Roasted Vegetables:
4 cups mixed vegetables (e.g., broccoli florets, bell peppers, carrots, snap peas)
2 tablespoons olive oil
Salt and pepper to taste
For the Peanut Sauce:
1/4 cup natural peanut butter

Two tablespoons tamari or soy sauce (for a gluten-free version)
2 tablespoons rice vinegar
1 tablespoon maple syrup or honey
1 clove garlic, minced
1 teaspoon grated fresh ginger
two to four tablespoons of warm water (adjust for consistency)
For the Stir Fry:
8 oz (about 225g) cooked and drained whole wheat noodles or rice (optional)

Chopped fresh cilantro and crushed peanuts for garnish (optional)
Lime wedges for serving (optional)

Roasting the Vegetables:
Preheat your oven to 425°F (220°C).
Combine salt, pepper, and olive oil with the mixed vegetables.
Place them in a single layer on a baking pan.

Roast the vegetables for 20 to 25 minutes or until they

are soft and have begun to caramelize,in a preheated oven. You can toss them once or twice during roasting for even cooking. Making the Peanut Sauce:

In a bowl, whisk together peanut butter, soy sauce or tamari, rice vinegar, maple syrup or honey, minced garlic, and grated ginger. Gradually add warm water, one tablespoon at a time, until you reach your desired sauce consistency. The warm water helps to thin out the peanut butter and make the sauce smooth.

Assembling the Stir Fry:
Cook the whole wheat noodles or rice according to package instructions, if using. Drain and set aside.

In a large skillet or wok, combine the roasted vegetables and cooked noodles or rice.

Pour the peanut sauce over the mixture and gently toss everything together until well coated and heated through.

Serve your roasted
vegetable stir fry with
peanut sauce hot,
garnished with chopped
fresh cilantro, crushed
peanuts, and lime wedges,
if desired.

CHAPTER THIRTEEN

Vegetables and Chickpea Salad
with Tahini Dressing:

For the Roasted
Vegetables:
4 cups mixed vegetables
(e.g., bell peppers, zucchini,
cherry tomatoes, red onion,
broccoli florets)
2 tablespoons olive oil
Salt and pepper to taste
1 teaspoon dried oregano
(optional)
For the Chickpeas:

One can (15 oz) of rinsed
and drained chickpeas
1 tablespoon olive oil
1/2 teaspoon smoked
paprika (or regular paprika)
Salt to taste
For the Tahini Dressing:
1/4 cup tahini
2 tablespoons lemon juice
2 tablespoons water (adjust
for desired consistency)
1 clove garlic, minced
1/2 teaspoon ground cumin
Salt and pepper to taste
For Garnish:

Fresh parsley or cilantro, chopped (optional)
Sesame seeds (optional)

Roasting the Vegetables:
Preheat your oven to 425°F (220°C).
Arrange the mixed vegetables on a baking sheet, cutting them into bite-sized pieces.
Drizzle with olive oil, season with salt, pepper, and dried oregano (if using), and toss to coat.
Roast the vegetables for 20 to 25 minutes until they are

soft and have a hint of caramelization,in a preheated oven. To ensure even cooking, stir or flip them halfway through.
Roasting the Chickpeas:
While the vegetables are roasting, in a separate small bowl, toss the drained and rinsed chickpeas with olive oil, smoked paprika, and a pinch of salt.
Spread the chickpeas on a separate baking sheet and roast in the same oven for about 15-20 minutes or until

they become crispy, shaking the pan occasionally.
Making the Tahini Dressing:
In a bowl, whisk together tahini, lemon juice, water, minced garlic, ground cumin, salt, and pepper until smooth. If necessary, thin the consistency with additional water.
Assembling the Salad:
Once the vegetables and chickpeas are roasted and slightly cooled, combine them in a large bowl.

Drizzle the tahini dressing over the roasted vegetables and chickpeas.
Gently toss everything together until well coated.
Garnish and Serve:
Garnish the salad with chopped fresh parsley or cilantro and sesame seeds, if desired.
Serve the Roasted Vegetable and Chickpea Salad with Tahini Dressing as a hearty and flavorful meal.
Enjoy this nutritious and satisfying salad with the

creamy tahini dressing and the crunch of roasted chickpeas!

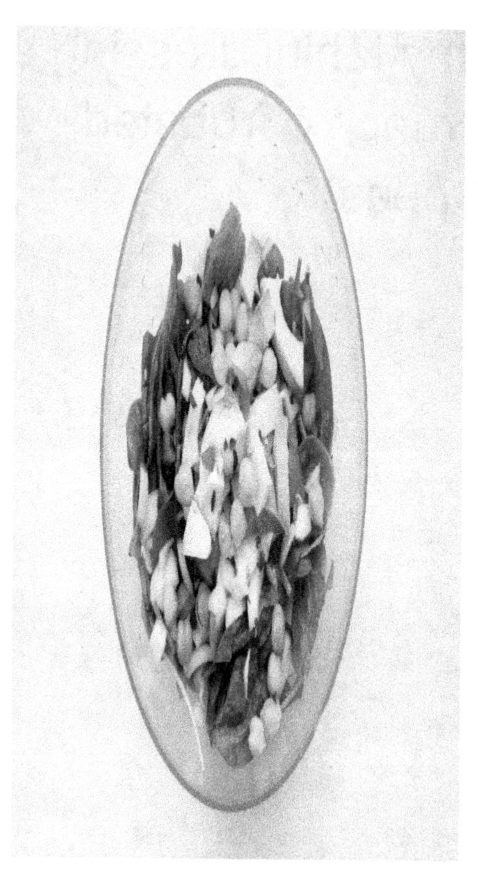

CHAPTER FOURTEEN

Lentil and Vegetable Curry with Coconut Milk:

For the Curry:
1 cup rinsed and drained dried lentils, either brown or green
1 onion, finely chopped
2 cloves garlic, minced
1 red bell pepper, diced
1 zucchini, diced
1 carrot, diced
1 can (14 oz) diced tomatoes
1 can (14 oz) coconut milk

2 tablespoons curry paste
(red, green, or yellow,
based on your preference
and spice level)
1 tablespoon vegetable oil
2 teaspoons curry powder
1 teaspoon ground turmeric
1 teaspoon ground cumin
Salt and pepper to taste
Fresh cilantro leaves for
garnish (optional)

Directions:

1. Cook the Lentils:
In a large saucepan,
combine the rinsed lentils
with 2.5 cups of water. Bring
to a boil, then reduce the

heat to low, cover, and simmer for about 20-25 minutes, or until the lentils are tender but not mushy. After draining, leave the cooked lentils aside.
2. Prepare the Curry:
In a large skillet or a wide pot, heat the vegetable oil over medium heat.
When the onion is transparent, add it and sauté it for two to three minutes.
Add the minced garlic, curry paste, curry powder, ground turmeric, and ground cumin.

Stir and cook for an additional 1-2 minutes to toast the spices and release their flavors.

Add the diced red bell pepper, zucchini, and carrot. The vegetables should start to soften after five to seven minutes of sautéing.

3. Simmer with Tomatoes and Coconut Milk:

Stir in the can of diced tomatoes and the can of coconut milk. Mix everything well.

Stir in the cooked lentils after adding them.

Bring the mixture to a gentle simmer and let it cook for about 10-15 minutes, allowing the flavors to meld together and the vegetables to become tender.
Season with salt and pepper to taste. Adjust the spice level by adding more curry paste if desired.
4. Serve:
Serve your Lentil and Vegetable Curry with Coconut Milk over cooked rice or with naan bread.
If desired, garnish with fresh cilantro leaves.

Enjoy this hearty and
flavorful lentil and vegetable
curry with the creamy
richness of coconut milk. It's
a comforting and nutritious
meal that's perfect for
vegetarians and vegans

CHAPTER FIFTEEN

Muesli Whole Grain with Berries
and Nuts:

Ingredients:

1 cup old-fashioned rolled
oats
2 cups water
Pinch of salt
Half a cup of mixed berries,
such as raspberries,
blueberries, and
strawberries
2 tablespoons chopped nuts
(e.g., almonds, walnuts, or
your favorite)
1 tablespoon honey or
maple syrup (optional)

1/2 teaspoon ground cinnamon (optional)
Milk or dairy-free milk alternative (e.g., almond milk, soy milk) for serving (optional)

Directions:

1. Cook the Oatmeal:

A small amount of salt, water, and rolled oats should all be combined in a medium pot.
Bring the mixture to a boil over medium-high heat, then reduce the heat to low and simmer for about 5-7

minutes, stirring occasionally.

Cook until the oatmeal reaches your desired level of thickness and creaminess. If you prefer a thicker oatmeal, cook for a shorter time. For a creamier consistency, cook for a bit longer.

2. Prepare the Toppings: While the oatmeal is cooking, wash and prepare the mixed berries. You can slice strawberries and leave smaller berries whole.

Chop the nuts of your choice if they are not already chopped.

3. Sweeten and Flavor (Optional):

Once the oatmeal is cooked to your liking, you can add optional ingredients for extra flavor. Stir in honey or maple syrup for sweetness and ground cinnamon for warmth. Adjust these to your taste preferences.

4. Serve:

Divide the cooked oatmeal into serving bowls.

Top each bowl with the mixed berries and chopped nuts.
If you prefer, you can drizzle a bit more honey or maple syrup over the toppings.
For added creaminess, you can pour a small amount of milk or dairy-free milk alternative over the oatmeal before serving.
5. Enjoy:
Your Whole Grain Oatmeal with Berries and Nuts is ready to enjoy! Dig in while it's warm for a comforting and nutritious breakfast.

This oatmeal recipe is versatile, and you can adjust it to suit your taste by adding other toppings like sliced bananas, chia seeds, or a dollop of yogurt. It's a healthy and fulfilling way to begin the day.

CHAPTER SIXTEEN

Tomato and Black Bean Taco Salad:

Ingredients:

For the Salad:
2 cups fresh mixed greens (e.g., lettuce, spinach)
1 cup cherry tomatoes, halved
One cup of rinsed and drained canned black beans
1 cup corn kernels (frozen, canned, or grilled)
1/2 red onion, finely chopped
1 avocado, diced

1/4 cup sliced black olives
(optional)
1 cup crushed tortilla chips
(optional)
For the Dressing:
1/4 cup olive oil
2 tablespoons lime juice
1 teaspoon chili powder
1/2 teaspoon cumin
1/2 teaspoon paprika
Salt and pepper to taste
For Garnish (optional):
Fresh cilantro, chopped
Shredded vegan cheese or
regular cheese (optional)

Vegan sour cream or regular sour cream (optional)

Directions:

1. Prepare the Dressing:

In a small bowl, whisk together the olive oil, lime juice, chili powder, cumin, paprika, salt, and pepper. Set aside.

2. Assemble the Salad:

In a large salad bowl, layer the mixed greens as the base.

Add the halved cherry tomatoes, drained black beans, corn kernels, finely chopped red onion, diced avocado, and sliced black olives (if using).

3. Toss and Dress: Drizzle the prepared dressing over the salad ingredients in the bowl. Toss everything together gently to coat all of the ingredients with the dressing.

4. Optional Additions: If desired, top the salad with crushed tortilla chips for extra crunch.

Garnish with chopped fresh cilantro and shredded

vegan cheese or regular
cheese.
Add a dollop of vegan sour
cream or regular sour
cream if you like.

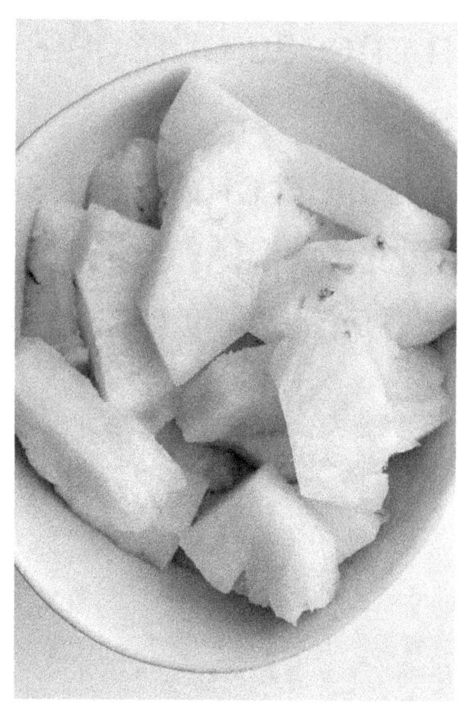

CHAPTER SEVENTEEN

Smoothies

 recipe for a Berry Blast
Smoothie:

Ingredients:
1 cup mixed berries (e.g.,
strawberries, blueberries,
raspberries, blackberries)
1/2 cup Greek yogurt (or
dairy-free yogurt if you're
vegan)
1 ripe banana
1 cup fresh spinach leaves
(optional for added nutrition)

1 tbsp chia seeds (optional for added fiber)

1/2 cup water or almond milk (adjust for desired thickness)

Honey or maple syrup for sweetness (optional)

Directions:

Prepare Your Ingredients:

Remove any stems or hulls from the mixed berries.

Peel the ripe banana.

Measure the Greek yogurt, chia seeds, and water or almond milk.

Blend the Ingredients:

In a blender, combine the mixed berries, banana, Greek yogurt, fresh spinach (if using), and chia seeds. Start blending on low speed and gradually increase to high until the mixture is smooth and well combined. If the smoothie is too thick, you can add water or almond milk a little at a time until it reaches your desired consistency.
Taste and Sweeten (if needed):

Taste the smoothie and add honey or maple syrup if you'd like it sweeter. This step is optional, as the natural sweetness of the fruits and yogurt may be sufficient.
Blend Again:

If you added sweetener, blend the smoothie again for a few seconds to incorporate it.
Serve:

Fill a glass halfway with your Berry Blast smoothie.

Garnish with extra berries, a sprinkle of chia seeds, or a slice of banana if desired. Enjoy:

Sip and enjoy your delicious and nutritious Berry Blast Smoothie! It's a refreshing and fiber-packed treat that's perfect for breakfast or a healthy snack.

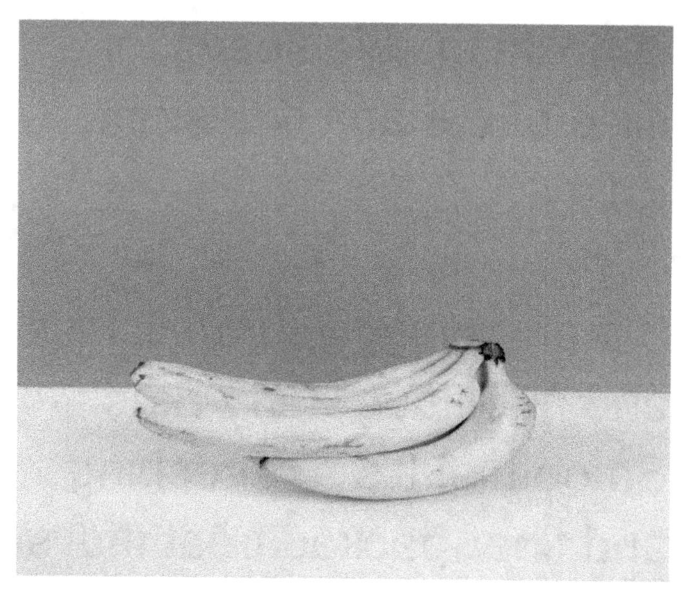

CHAPTER EIGHTEEN

Recipe for a Green Power Smoothie:

Ingredients:

1 cup fresh spinach leaves

1 cup kale leaves, stems removed

1 ripe banana

1 cup diced pineapple (fresh or frozen)

1 cup almond milk (or your choice of milk)

1 tablespoon ground flaxseeds (optional, for added fiber and omega-3)

Honey or maple syrup for sweetness (optional)

Directions:
Prepare Your Ingredients:
Thoroughly wash the fresh spinach and kale leaves.
Peel the ripe banana.
Dice the pineapple if using fresh pineapple.
Blend the Ingredients:
In a blender, add the fresh spinach leaves, kale leaves, ripe banana, diced pineapple, and ground flaxseeds (if using).
Pour in the almond milk.
Blend Until Smooth:
Begin by blending in low and gradually increase to

high. Blend until smooth and all of the ingredients are well combined.
Taste and Sweeten (if needed):
Taste the Green Power Smoothie and add honey or maple syrup if you'd like it sweeter. This step is optional, as the natural sweetness of the banana and pineapple may be sufficient.
Blend Again (if sweetened):

If you added sweetener, blend the smoothie again

for a few seconds to incorporate it.
Serve:
Fill a glass with your Green Power Smoothie.
Sip and enjoy your nutritious Green Power Smoothie! It's packed with vitamins, minerals, and fiber, making it a great choice for a healthy and energizing drink.
You can also add ice cubes if you prefer a colder smoothie, or a scoop of protein powder for an extra boost of protein.

CHAPTER NINETEEN

Recipe for a Tropical Paradise
Smoothie:

Ingredients:

1 cup diced mango (fresh or
frozen)
1 cup diced papaya (fresh
or frozen)
1/2 cup canned coconut
milk (adjust to taste and
consistency)
½ cup Greek yoghurt (or
dairy-free yoghurt if you're
vegan)
1tbsp shredded coconut
(plus additional for garnish)

1/4 teaspoon ground turmeric (optional, for color and flavor)

Honey or maple syrup for sweetness (optional)

Directions:

Prepare Your Ingredients:

Peel and dice the mango and papaya.

Measure the coconut milk, Greek yogurt, shredded coconut, and ground turmeric (if using).

Blend the Ingredients:

In a blender, combine the diced mango, diced papaya, coconut milk, Greek yogurt,

shredded coconut, and ground turmeric (if using).
Blend Until Smooth:
Begin by blending on low and gradually increase to high. Blend untill smooth and all of the ingredients are well combined.
Taste and Sweeten (if needed):
Taste the Tropical Paradise Smoothie and add honey or maple syrup if you'd like it sweeter. This step is optional, as the natural sweetness of the mango

and papaya may be
sufficient.
Blend Again (if sweetened):
If you added sweetener,
blend the smoothie again
for a few seconds to
incorporate it.
Serve:
Pour your Tropical Paradise
Smoothie into a glass.
Garnish (optional):
Garnish your smoothie with
additional shredded coconut
for a tropical touch.

Sip and enjoy your
refreshing and
tropical-inspired smoothie!

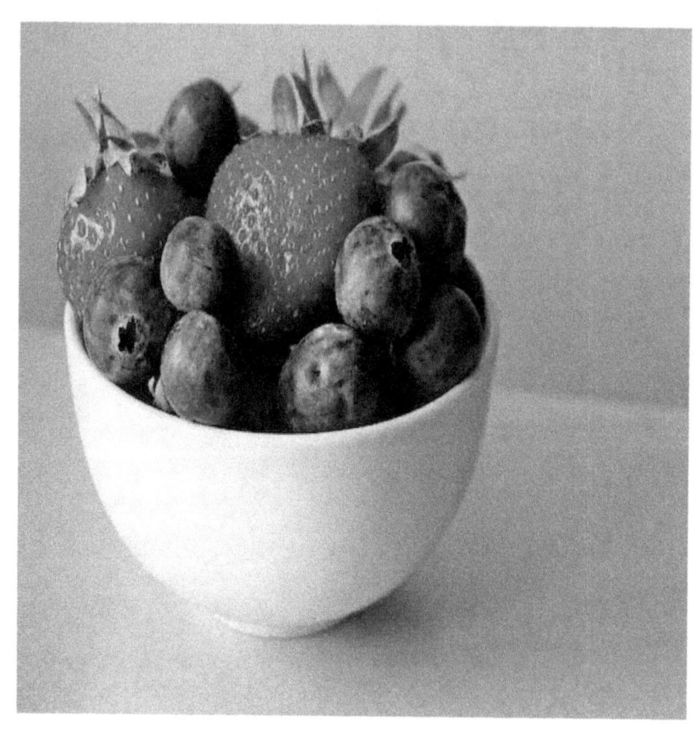

CHAPTER TWENTY

simple and delicious recipe for a
Peanut Butter Banana Smoothie:

Ingredients:

2 ripe bananas
2 tablespoons peanut butter
(natural peanut butter
without added sugar is a
healthy choice)
1/2 cup rolled oats
1 1/2 cups milk (dairy milk,
almond milk, or your
preferred milk)
1 tbsp honey or maple
syrup (optional, for added
sweetness)
1/2 teaspoon vanilla extract

A handful of ice cubes
(optional)

Directions:

Prepare Your Ingredients:
Peel and cut the ripe
bananas into smaller
chunks.

Measure the peanut butter,
rolled oats, milk, honey or
maple syrup (if using), and
vanilla extract.

Blend the Ingredients:
In a blender, add the
banana chunks, peanut
butter, rolled oats, milk,
honey or maple syrup (if
using), and vanilla extract.

If you like your smoothie extra cold, you can also add a handful of ice cubes.
Blend Until Smooth:
Begin by blending on low and gradually increase to high. Blend until the mixture is smooth and well combined.
Taste and Adjust (if needed):
Taste the Peanut Butter Banana Smoothie and adjust the sweetness by adding more honey or maple syrup if desired. Blend briefly to incorporate.

Serve:

Fill a glass halfway with Peanut Butter Banana Smoothie.

Sip and enjoy your creamy and nutty Peanut Butter Banana Smoothie! It's a satisfying and protein-rich drink that's perfect for breakfast or a snack.

Feel free to customize this recipe by adding a handful of spinach or kale for extra greens or a scoop of protein powder for added protein. Enjoy!

CHAPTER TWENTY-ONE

Recipe for a Chocolate Avocado
Smoothie:

Ingredients:

1 ripe avocado, peeled and
pitted
2 tablespoons unsweetened
cocoa powder
1 cup almond milk (or other
milk of choice)
2 tablespoons honey or
maple syrup (adjust for
sweetness)
1/2 teaspoon vanilla extract
A pinch of salt
Ice cubes (optional for a
colder smoothie)

Directions:
Prepare Your Ingredients:
Peel and pit the ripe
avocado.
Blend the Ingredients:
In a blender, combine the
peeled avocado,
unsweetened cocoa
powder, almond milk, honey
or maple syrup (adjust for
sweetness), vanilla extract,
and a pinch of salt.
Blend Until Smooth:
Begin by blending on low
and gradually increase to
high. Blend until the mixture

is smooth and well combined.
Taste and Adjust (if needed):
Taste the Chocolate Avocado Smoothie and adjust the sweetness by adding more honey or maple syrup if desired.
Blend briefly to incorporate.
Serve:
Pour your Chocolate Avocado Smoothie into a glass.
Sip and enjoy your rich and creamy Chocolate Avocado

Smoothie! It's a delightful and nutritious treat.

This smoothie is not only delicious but also a great way to enjoy the healthy fats and nutrients from avocados. Feel free to customize it by adding a dash of cinnamon or a spoonful of Greek yogurt for extra creaminess if you like. Enjoy your chocolaty indulgence.

CHAPTER TWENTY-TWO

Recipe for a Chia Berry Smoothie:

Ingredients:

1 cup berries (strawberries, blueberries, raspberries, etc.)
1/2 cup Greek yoghurt (or dairy-free yoghurt if you're vegan)
1 banana
1 tablespoon chia seeds
1/2 cup almond milk (or other milk of choice)
Honey or maple syrup for sweetness (optional)

Ice cubes (optional for a colder smoothie)

Directions:

Prepare Your Ingredients:

Wash the mixed berries if needed.

Peel the banana.

Blend the Ingredients:

In a blender, combine the mixed berries, Greek yogurt, banana, chia seeds, almond milk, and honey or maple syrup (if using).

Blend Until Smooth:

Begin by blending on low and gradually increase to high. Blend until the mixture

is smooth and well combined.
Taste and Adjust (if needed):
Taste the Chia Berry Smoothie and adjust the sweetness by adding more honey or maple syrup if desired. Blend briefly to incorporate.
Serve:
Pour your Chia Berry Smoothie into a glass.
Sip and enjoy your fruity and fiber-rich Chia Berry Smoothie! It's a refreshing and nutritious drink that's

perfect for breakfast or a snack.

Feel free to customize this recipe by adding other fruits or a scoop of protein powder for added protein. Chia seeds add a nice texture and an extra dose of fiber and omega-3 fatty acids to your smoothie. Enjoy!

CHAPTER TWENTY-THREE

Recipe for a Pineapple Spinach Smoothie:

Ingredients:

1 cup fresh spinach leaves

1 1/2 cups diced pineapple (fresh or frozen)

1/2 cup Greek yogurt (or dairy free yogurt if you're vegan)

1/2 cup coconut water

1 tablespoon flaxseeds (optional, for added fiber and omega-3)

Honey or maple syrup for sweetness (optional)

Ice cubes (optional for a colder smoothie)

Directions:

Prepare Your Ingredients:

Wash the fresh spinach leaves.

Dice the pineapple if using fresh pineapple.

Blend the Ingredients:

In a blender, add the fresh spinach leaves, diced pineapple, Greek yogurt, coconut water, and flaxseeds (if using).

Blend Until Smooth:

Begin by blending on low and gradually increase to

high. Blend until the mixture is smooth and well combined.

Taste and Adjust (if needed):

Taste the Pineapple Spinach Smoothie and adjust the sweetness by adding honey or maple syrup if desired. Blend briefly to incorporate.

Serve:

Pour your Pineapple Spinach Smoothie into a glass.

Sip and enjoy your tropical and nutrient-packed

Pineapple Spinach
Smoothie! It's a refreshing
and healthy drink.
Feel free to customize this
recipe by adding a squeeze
of lime juice for extra
tanginess or a scoop of
protein powder for added
protein. The combination of
pineapple and spinach
creates a deliciously sweet
and vibrant green smoothie
that's both tasty and
nutritious. Enjoy!

CHAPTER TWENTY-FOUR

Recipe for a Kiwi Kale Smoothie:

Ingredients:

2 ripe kiwis, peeled and sliced

1 cup fresh kale leaves, stems removed

1 banana

1/2 cup orange juice (freshly squeezed or store-bought)

1/2 cup Greek yoghurt (or dairy-free yoghurt if you're vegan)

Honey or maple syrup for sweetness (optional)

Ice cubes (optional for a colder smoothie)
Directions:
Prepare Your Ingredients:
Peel and slice the ripe kiwis.
Wash the fresh kale leaves and remove the stems.
Peel the banana.
Blend the Ingredients:
In a blender, add the sliced kiwis, fresh kale leaves, banana, orange juice, Greek yogurt, and honey or maple syrup (if using).
Blend Until Smooth:

Begin by blending on low
and gradually increase to
high. Blend until the mixture
is smooth and well
combined.
Taste and Adjust (if
needed):
Taste the Kiwi Kale
Smoothie and adjust the
sweetness by adding honey
or maple syrup if desired.
Blend briefly to incorporate.
Serve:
Pour your Kiwi Kale
Smoothie into a glass.

Sip and enjoy your vibrant and vitamin-packed Kiwi Kale Smoothie! It's a refreshing and nutritious green drink.
Feel free to customize this recipe by adding a squeeze of lemon juice for extra zing or a handful of frozen mango for a tropical twist. Kale and kiwi make a fantastic combination, providing a burst of color and health benefits to your smoothie. Enjoy

CHAPTER TWENTY-FIVE

Recipe for a Mango Carrot Smoothie:

Ingredients:

1 cup diced mango (fresh or frozen)

1 large carrot, peeled and chopped

1/2 cup Greek yoghurt (or dairy-free yoghurt if you're vegan)

1/2 cup coconut water (or your choice of milk)

1 tbsp honey or maple syrup (optional, for added sweetness)

A squeeze of lime juice
(optional, for added zing)
Ice cubes (optional for a
colder smoothie)
Directions:
Prepare Your Ingredients:
Dice the mango if using
fresh mango.
Peel and chop the carrot.
Blend the Ingredients:
In a blender, combine the
diced mango, chopped
carrot, Greek yogurt,
coconut water, and honey or
maple syrup (if using).
Blend Until Smooth:

Begin by blending on low
and gradually increase to
high. Blend until the mixture
is smooth and well
combined.
Taste and Adjust (if
needed):
Taste the Mango Carrot
Smoothie and adjust the
sweetness by adding honey
or maple syrup if desired.
For added flavor, squeeze
in a little lime juice.
Pour your Mango Carrot
Smoothie into a glass.
Sip and enjoy your sunny
and nutritious Mango Carrot

Smoothie! It's a delicious way to enjoy the sweetness of mango and the goodness of carrots.

Feel free to customize this recipe by adding a pinch of ground ginger for a spicy kick or a tablespoon of chia seeds for added fiber.

Mango and carrot create a delightful combination of flavors and vibrant color in this smoothie. Enjoy

CHAPTER TWENTY-SIX

Recipe for a Blueberry Almond Smoothie:

Ingredients:

1 cup fresh or frozen blueberries
1/4 cup almonds (unsalted)
1 cup fresh spinach leaves (optional for added nutrition)
1 cup almond milk (or other milk of choice)
1 tbsp honey or maple syrup (optional, for added sweetness)
Ice cubes (optional for a colder smoothie)
Directions:

Prepare Your Ingredients:
If using fresh blueberries,
rinse them.
Measure the almonds, fresh
spinach leaves (if using),
almond milk, honey or
maple syrup (if using).
Blend the Ingredients:
In a blender, add the
blueberries, almonds, fresh
spinach leaves (if using),
almond milk, and honey or
maple syrup (if using).
Blend Until Smooth:
Begin by blending on low
and gradually increase to
high. Blend until the mixture

is smooth and well combined.

Taste and Adjust (if needed):

Taste the Blueberry Almond Smoothie and adjust the sweetness by adding honey or maple syrup if desired.

Serve:

Pour your Blueberry Almond Smoothie into a glass.

Sip and enjoy your antioxidant-rich and nutritious Blueberry Almond Smoothie! It's a delightful and healthy drink.

Feel free to customize this recipe by adding a teaspoon of almond butter for extra nutty flavor or a scoop of protein powder for added protein. Blueberries and almonds create a fantastic combination of flavors and provide a burst of health benefits in this smoothie. Enjoy

CONCLUSION

In conclusion, the Fiber Fueled Cookbook for Beginners is a gateway to a healthier, more vibrant lifestyle. Through its pages, we've explored the incredible benefits of fiber-rich foods and the impact they can have on our overall well-being. By embracing this dietary approach, you're not just choosing a cookbook; you're choosing a path to improved health, increased energy, and a stronger connection with the planet.

This cookbook is not just about recipes; it's a journey towards a sustainable and delicious way of eating. We've uncovered the power of whole grains, legumes, fruits, and vegetables to transform our bodies from the inside out. Whether you're seeking weight management, better digestion, or enhanced heart health, this cookbook has you covered.

We've learned how to prepare mouthwatering dishes that cater to diverse tastes and dietary needs, making it accessible to everyone. It's a celebration of the abundance of plant-based ingredients, the joy of experimentation in the kitchen, and the pleasure of savoring every bite.

With the Fiber Fueled Cookbook for Beginners,

you're not just changing the way you eat; you're changing your life. Here's to a future filled with vibrant health, culinary adventures, and a newfound appreciation for the remarkable world of fiber-rich foods. Bon appétit